Autobiography of an Agoraphobic

One Man's Struggle With Panic Disorder

By

Michael R. Patrick

This book is a work of non-fiction. Names and places have been changed to protect the privacy of all individuals. The events and situations are true.

ISBN: 1-4107-8629-3 (e-book)
ISBN: 1-4107-8630-7 (Paperback)

This book is printed on acid free paper.

1stBooks – rev. 01/04/06

Dedication

I would like to dedicate this book, and all books to come, God willing, to my wife, Mary without whom this book could not have been written.

I also commemorate this book to the late Joseph Cardinal Bernardin of Chicago, and the late Mother Téresa of Calcutta, and also to the late Pope John Paul II for their inspiration in writing this book.

In The Love of God

Michael R. Patrick

Michael R. Patrick

Table of Contents

Chapter 1

"I am poured out like water, and all my bones are out of joint: My Heart has

become like wax; melting away in my bosom" - Psalm 22:14

Imagine that you are in a plane at 30,000 feet. Suddenly two men start to pull you toward the door. Then a third man opens up the door. As the two men pull you closer your fear is building. You know something terrible is going to happen. When you get to the door of the plane, the three men push you out. You're falling, and you know when you hit the ground you will die. You start screaming, but no one can help you. You continue to fall, and fall, and fall, but you never hit the ground. You are in a perpetual, terrifying fear, and you know it will never end. You can't breathe, your heart is racing, and it will never stop.

If you can imagine how you would feel if this event happened to you, then you could get the idea of what a panic attack is like. My name is Michael Patrick. I live in the Midwest, a suburb of the largest city in the state. I have experienced the above event several hundred times in the 24 years I've had agoraphobia with panic disorder. I'm 49 years old, I'm Catholic, and by the time I was 30 years old I had been hospitalized for my condition three times. I'm writing this book because I want other people to know my story, and how God saw me through a living nightmare. I want to give hope to those who have panic disorder, and to enlighten those who don't. Since I led a fairly ordinary life until I was 19, I will begin my story there, at the age of 19, when I had my first panic attack.

In 1973, at the age of 19, I was attending college at a large state university in the Midwest. I was a normal college student who was very intelligent and tended to be a perfectionist. I had recently had my tonsils out the year before, and a short time after I had contracted mononucleosis, which I had for almost six months, causing me to miss the second semester of my freshman year. Just before returning to start my second year of college, I had contracted a virus, which caused me to have fatigue, loss of appetite, and a low-grade temperature. I went to college still sick, in the hope that I would soon be well again. Unfortunately, this was not to be the case. Two days later, with a temperature of 103°, I went to the University health center, which misdiagnosed my illness as a cold. The doctor ran no tests, nor did he do a physical examination. All he did was look at my throat and told me to rest for a few days. I went back to my dormitory and I was so sick I didn't leave my dorm for two days. My friends on the floor brought food from the cafeteria to me. Since I wasn't getting any help from the doctor at the university, I called my own doctor, who was 50 miles away, and made an appointment. The day before the appointment I felt somewhat better, so I went into the recreation room to watch TV with some friends. All of a sudden, I felt as if I couldn't breathe. I inhaled more, and breathed deeper, but the sensation never went away. I said to my friends, "I can't breathe!" Then it got worse. I was taken to the emergency room of the local hospital, and the nurse on call told me I was hyperventilating. I thought certainly I would die. She gave me a shot of tranquilizer, which helped, but not much. For two hours in the emergency room I hyperventilated. I thought almost certainly I would die, but never did. My friends drove me to my hometown hospital, where I was admitted for tests. My doctor discovered that my liver was enlarged and tender, and after doing some blood tests he discovered that I had walked off a case of severe viral hepatitis, and he told me later that I could have died from it. He told me I was in no danger now; but I was still having attacks of hyperventilation, and the only advice I received was to breathe into a paper bag each time it occurred. This, however, never relieved the terror I had experienced, a terror that haunts me even to this day.

I was told I needed to see a psychiatrist, because in addition to the problem of hyperventilation, I had become very depressed from all that I had gone through, and had lost 30 pounds due to having no appetite for food. I was convinced that I had a heart problem, but my doctor could not find anything wrong with my heart, after listening to it and giving me an EKG. Many years later I would find out he was wrong, but since at the time everything pointed to a psychiatric problem, he recommended that I see a psychiatrist. So I made an appointment with a local psychiatrist, and this began my long road back to being normal and functioning, a road that did not come to an end until recently.

Chapter 2

"My God, my God, why have you forsaken me? Why art thou so far from helping me, and from the words of my cry?"- Psalm 22:1

I met Dr. Lupek (a pseudonym), a local psychiatrist, about a month after I came home from the local hospital. He was a big man, about 6 feet tall, overweight, and about 50 years old, who smoked cigarettes one after another. During my first visit he told that I had depression, and that it was caused by a chemical imbalance that was causing my fear, and he said he wanted to put me on medication, but I refused. I did not want to be dependent on a pill to keep me functioning. He said that I would probably do okay without medication, and he decided to treat my depression and anxiety with psychotherapy. He never once mentioned that I could have agoraphobia.

I saw Dr. Lupek for about six months, and then decided that I wanted to return to college. I went back to the same state university whose health center misdiagnosed my viral hepatitis as a cold. This was a big mistake. I was under a psychiatrist's care and then went away to school 50 miles from home. I lived in a dorm, which was extremely noisy, and there were racial tensions at the whole school. In fact, two windows on my floor had bullet holes in them from a sniper shooting into rooms at random. I decided I would finish the semester and then transfer to a Catholic University in the City. In the meantime, Dr. Lupek had placed me on 2 mg of Stelazine for my anxiety, and it helped somewhat, but not much. One Saturday, as I was watching TV, some of my friends had gotten together to play softball, and asked if I wanted to play. I was a good athlete and liked to play softball, so I took them up on their invitation. During the game, I was sliding into second base, when I hit a rock in the base path with my right knee. As it turned out, I ended up tearing a cartilage in that knee, and at the end of the semester, in my hometown hospital, I had it operated on.

The night before the surgery I felt tremendous fear. Ever since I hyperventilated a year before, I had developed a grave dread of hospitals, and especially of death. At that time, my faith in Christ was not strong enough to overcome my fear of death, because I suffered from panic disorder at the time and didn't know it. I can even to this day remember the first time I hyperventilated, laying on my back, looking up at the ceiling of the emergency room for my heart to stop beating. This was the same fear I had when I was wheeled into the emergency room for my knee surgery. Even though I had been given a large dose of Demerol, I was still panicking as they made preparations for me to go under the anesthetic. The last thing I remember before going unconscious was begging the anesthesiologist to knock me out so I would stop hyperventilating. You see, when you have panic disorder, the fear of death never leaves you. It is a haunting specter waiting to rear its terrifying head at any moment, and there's nothing you can do to stop it.

The surgery itself went well, however the surgeon failed to have me lift weights after the operation. My knee was weak, but I did not have any pain. I transferred to a Catholic University in the City and started school there in April of 1985. I took the train then walked a mile and a half to the campus. I liked the school tremendously, and did very well my first quarter, with straight A's in all of my classes. I continued doing very well for a year, and decided I would major in Finance, since I loved mathematics and Finance was heavy math. I also made a lot of friends at the Catholic University, and developed an active social life on the weekends, but still remained firmly committed to my studies during the week.

Then one day disaster struck. I was late for my train and was running down the stairs from the 4th floor of the University. I put most of my weight on my left knee, because my right knee was weak, when suddenly I felt a sharp pain in my left knee. The pain continued to increase as I walked down the stairs. By the time I got to street level, I could hardly walk due to the pain. I went to the same orthopedic surgeon who operated on my right knee, and he diagnosed it as a torn cartilage and said I needed surgery. In March of 1976, he operated on my left knee. Instead of a torn cartilage, I had a torn anterior cruciate ligament, and loose cartilage. He repaired the ligament, but left the cartilage in, in the hope it would tighten. Unfortunately for me, it did not, and instead became torn. In August 1976, I had my left knee operated on, but this time I had a different surgeon from the same hospital. As usual, I experienced the same terrible fear being wheeled into the

7

operating room, and had a panic attack even though I was heavily sedated with Demerol. This surgeon discovered that not just the outside cartilage was torn, but the inside cartilage was torn also, and the underside of my kneecap had to be shaved to remove irregularities. The technical name for this is chondromalacia of the patella. I woke up from the operation in the most pain I had ever experienced. It felt as if someone had hit me in my knee with a baseball bat. But this was only the start of my troubles. The surgery was largely unsuccessful, and as a result I was in pain almost constantly.

I returned back to the Catholic University in the City in September of 1976 and started taking classes again. I was leaving class one spring evening with a friend of mine. We walked toward a parking garage near school, because he was going to give me a ride to the train station. I remember waiting at a traffic light and looking up at the stars. All of a sudden, the thought of the vast openness of space hit me, and I started to feel like I was falling. I felt dizzy, disoriented, and had trouble breathing. This was the onset of agoraphobia, but I was not to find that out until three years later. I shook off the sensation after a few minutes and went home. I went to bed that night with a strange foreboding of future problems, but I brushed it off as only anxiety, and finally went to sleep.

I went to school the next morning and on my walk to school I experienced the same frightening sensation I had experienced the night before, only this time it wouldn't go away. For some reason, instinctively, I knew I had to ground myself, to bring myself back to being in contact with solid earth again. I reached out and grabbed the nearest post, and held on tightly, shaking in fear. I held on as if for dear life itself, not daring to let go until the sensation had passed. I knew I was making a fool of myself in front of the people passing by, who looked at me wondering what was wrong with me, but I didn't care. I thought I was going to die, and it didn't matter to me what other people thought of me. If they thought I was weird, so be it. All I cared about was dealing with the attack I was experiencing. (Now you know why they call it a panic <u>attack</u>, because that's exactly what it is. It assaults you suddenly and without warning with an all-encompassing overpowering terror.) After the panic attack was over, I felt drained, but continued walking to the university, and completed the rest of the day and came home.

The next day I saw Dr. Lupek and told him what happened. He said I should take 20 milligrams of valium per day and just forget about it. He said I had a lot of fears, but was common in someone suffering from a biochemical depression. I continued with school, and over the next few months I experienced a panic attack almost daily. I kept informing Dr. Lupek of this, but never once did he mention the word agoraphobia. I told him the Valium was not helping, and at this point I was concerned that it may not be a mental problem at all, but something horrible like a brain tumor or a heart disease. He dismissed everything as anxiety, told me to quit complaining, and get on with life. At one point, when he was telling me something totally off the wall, I interrupted and said to him "yes, But...". He got angry with me and sarcastically told me I was suffering from the "Yes, But" syndrome. He knew I thought he was a quack, which was what he was. The only reason I stayed with him is that I didn't know of any other psychiatrist I could use. He had a monopoly in the town I was in. Anyway, I continued going to college, and things kept getting worse. At one point, while I was walking from school to the train station, I had to literally run from street lamp to street lamp and grab on, all the while praying to God to not let me die. I had even gone as far as to be afraid of gravity stopping and me falling up into the large open sky, an agoraphobic's worst nightmare.

As a result of the almost constant fear of open spaces, I had to stop taking the train to school, because I could not walk the 1 ½ miles from the train station to the university's campus, so I began driving to school. Fortunately for me, there was a parking garage about 100 feet from the campus, which allowed me to get to school and avoid the painful fear-ridden trek to and from the train station. But my reprieve did not last long. You see, with agoraphobia and with panic disorder, you gradually start to limit yourself to "safe places". The overall, main feeling in my case was a sensation of being "trapped" in an open space from which I could not escape. For the person who does not know about agoraphobia, I could liken the sensation as being the same as when a person with claustrophobia is locked in a tiny box just big enough to hold his body. The claustrophobic feels the panic, the absolute necessity of "getting out". For the agoraphobic, the opposite is true. The agoraphobic's main objective is "getting inside" somewhere to escape the open space. Only that will relieve his anxiety. In the beginning, for me the inside of my car was a "safe" place,

10

but that gradually began to change. The expressway started to become frightening. I began to think, what if I had a panic attack on the highway? Would I lose control of the car and kill myself and maybe someone else? So now, I had constant fear while driving the 20 miles from my home to the university, and gradually I started to fear even leaving the house. This forced me to cut back on my classes and go to school only 3 days a week. Surprisingly enough, during this entire mental trauma, I was still able to hold a 3.62 out of 4.0 grade point average. I don't know how I did it. Perhaps it was just will power, because I was even getting panic attacks in class. I would hold on to the desk while sitting in it and silently suffer. I was begging God everyday to help me. I wished I were dead, but never thought of killing myself because I was too afraid of death. What if I died and in the next life I was stuck in an open space all alone for all eternity? It was a thought almost too frightening to think, but it haunted me everyday, and I was only 23 years old.

Well, as you would probably guess, I withdrew from college in 1978, just four courses short of a degree. I just couldn't do it anymore. I decided I would try to get work somewhere, doing anything, which would enable me to survive. My parents were not rich, and I couldn't live off them, so I had to find work. However, there was a major economic recession at the time, and finding work was like pulling teeth. I became more and more depressed as my job search proved fruitless. Gradually, I started to go out of the house less and less, and the fear kept getting greater and greater. After six months I was almost totally homebound. I was too afraid to venture outside the house. I even got so bad that I could only come out of my room to eat and shower. The rest of the time I lay in bed, holding onto the bedpost, terrified and crippled with fear. I didn't know what was wrong with me, and I began to think I could have a brain tumor. Dr. Lupek was absolutely useless and incompetent, and he didn't help me at all. All the signs and symptoms of agoraphobia were there, and he never saw it, because he didn't even know such a disease existed. He was a total fool, and for two years I suffered with agoraphobia and panic attacks daily, sometimes several times a day, and he was too stupid to diagnose it and treat it. He didn't know what was wrong with me, so he wanted to hospitalize me, and the last thing I wanted was him taking care of me. I had lost 30 pounds and now only weighed 140 pounds, and I'm 6 feet tall. I really thought I was going to die. I knew I needed to get away from Lupek, and I decided to go to a teaching hospital in the City, which had an excellent reputation in just about every field of medicine. This was my last chance, it seemed, and things looked very bad for me.

But God was watching over me, and He did not abandon me, even though at the time I thought He had. Things were to get better in the near future, for God is good, and He will not allow evil except that greater good will come of it. Romans 8:28 says, "We know that God makes all things work together for the good of those who have been called according to His decree". This is so true. In December of 1979, at the age of 25, I went by ambulance to the teaching hospital in the City. This was to be the start of my healing, a slow and gradual one, but a healing nonetheless.

Chapter 3

"He relied on the Lord, let Him deliver him: let Him rescue him, if He loves him."

-Psalm 22:9

When I arrived at the hospital I was put on a medical floor, because the doctor that admitted me, Dr. Chan, was not a psychiatrist but an orthopedic surgeon, and also because he suspected some physical disease. (He was the orthopedic surgeon from which I had gotten a second opinion on my knees' conditions. He had said I would recover but the surgeons at the local hospital where I had the surgery had almost crippled me.) He ordered a CAT scan of my brain, and called in a neurologist to examine me. Dr. Doyle, the neurologist, told me that I had a 1% chance of having a tumor at the base of my brainstem. He also ordered an EEG to see if I had any abnormalities in my brain waves. However, I was not able to leave my hospital room due to the fear I had. I was lying on my bed with my hand tightly clenched holding onto the bed rail. I had constant fear. Dr. Chan sent in a young psychiatrist named Dr. Cocoran, and Dr. Cocoran gently told me that I had agoraphobia, and that there were medications that would help me. At last my problems had a name! How good God is! I talked with Dr. Cocoran briefly, and was impressed with his knowledge and his brilliant mind. In addition to this, he treated me like a human being, not like an animal as Dr. Lupek had done. Dr.

Cocoran had compassion and was kind to me. At first I didn't trust him, because dealing with Dr. Lupek had turned me off on all doctors, but gradually I came to realize his concern for me was genuine. He told me there was a medication called Imipramine with which he wanted to try to treat my agoraphobia. I welcomed the opportunity to get some relief from the paralyzing fear I was in. He mentioned that it would be easier to treat me on the psychiatric ward, and that it would be easier for me to take the brain scan and the EEG once the medication started to work. It sounded like a good idea to me, and so I agreed to be transferred to the psychiatric ward.

Two attendants came and wheeled me on a gurney into the psychiatric ward. It wasn't anything like I expected it to be. There were manic-depressives, schizophrenics, the severely depressed, and elderly people with less serious problems who were just moderately depressed. Some people also had physical ailments such as diabetes and heart disease, accompanying their depression or anxiety. But we all had one thing in common, we were not severe psychiatric cases, just moderate ones. The severe people were treated on another wing of the hospital.

The staff was very nice to me, but it was still no fun. It wasn't Disneyland, but it wasn't Hell either. I had only one problem, and that was the way the floor was laid out. The patient rooms were down long narrow corridors, and there was a large open area where the cafeteria was. This posed big problems for an agoraphobic. Being inside long, narrow corridors is a nightmare for someone with severe agoraphobia, as is eating in a large open space. For the last two years I had been unable to even sit in a fast food restaurant, so it was a nightmare trying to eat in a cafeteria. Often I would have to bring my food back into my room to eat, because I was getting panic attacks in the cafeteria. I soon found out that being in a psychiatric ward was no fun. It's noisy, very depressing, and everyone is suffering greatly. But here I was, so I decided to make the best of it.

Dr. Cocoran started to treat me with Imipramine. At the time, in 1979, there were only two drugs approved to treat agoraphobia. One was Imipramine, the other was Nardil. Nardil had dietary restrictions and was much harder to take, so Dr. Cocoran decided to try Imipramine first. Imipramine was not easy to take. It made my heart beat 140 beats per minute, I was severely constipated, I was dizzy, and my mouth was constantly parched and as dry as a desert. However, it did help somewhat with the panic attacks and agoraphobia, and I was finally able to take the CAT scan and the EEG which had been ordered by Dr. Doyle. Both were completely normal, and I breathed a sigh of relief.

Dr. Cocoran explained to me what agoraphobia was. The word "agora" is the Greek word for "marketplace" and "phobia" is "fear". So the word agoraphobia literally means "fear of the marketplace". But you have to remember what a marketplace was like in ancient Greece. It was a large open space crowded with people, and open spaces are what agoraphobic's dread. The reason they fear open spaces is because open space triggers a panic attack, a sudden onslaught of paralyzing fear, which causes you to feel like you are going to die. So, in reality, the agoraphobic really fears the panic attack the most. The fear associated with agoraphobia is multifaceted. It includes a fear of elevators, escalators, shopping malls (especially large malls which are enclosed), restaurants, bridges, and driving on expressways. Dr. Cocoran explained to me that the anxiety associated with agoraphobia and panic attacks can cause a person to have chest pain, sweating, dizziness, shortness of breath, and it can even make the agoraphobic seem as if things are not real. I think the last symptom is what causes agoraphobics who have panic attacks to feel like they're "going crazy". Dr. Cocoran even told me that some agoraphobics have had needless, unnecessary cardiac angiograms because they are convinced that the chest pain they have is a symptom of coronary artery disease. A panic attack can often mimic the symptoms of a heart attack, and that is why the angiograms are performed. He also told me that agoraphobia with panic disorder is a symptom of a biochemical imbalance in one's brain. It was not an emotional problem, it was a physical disease of my brain, and it was affecting my mind. He explained to me that there are two types of depression; one is a biochemical depression, and the other is a psychological depression. A biochemical depression is treated with medication, and that's why I was on Imipramine. A psychological depression is treated with psychotherapy and prayer. (Yes, you heard me right, I said a prayer. Dr. Cocoran, as it turns out, was a Christian.) What caused my agoraphobia? As it turned out, heredity played a part, but the stress incurred from my knee operations, and the mono, and the hepatitis also helped trigger the agoraphobia, along with the main reason for the panic disorder, which will be revealed in a later chapter of this book.

So, the main benefit of being hospitalized was that I gained tremendous knowledge about my disease, and that, for the first time in two years, gave me hope. I was discharged from the hospital after six weeks, and I continued to take the Imipramine for my agoraphobia. However, after a few months I had to discontinue it because the side effects, for me, became intolerable. Most other people tolerate Imipramine quite well, but I did not. I was afraid that all the hope I had was in vain, but God was not through with me yet. My Lord would not let me down.

Chapter 4

"I am the resurrection and the life, whoever believes in me, even though he die shall live and he who believes in me shall never die."- John 11:25

When Dr. Cocoran knew that I could no longer take the Imipramine he took me off it, and then he placed me on Nardil. Nardil is another antidepressant like Imipramine, but in a different class of drugs called "monoamine oxidase inhibitors", or MAO Inhibitors for short. MAO Inhibitors can be difficult to take, because they can have life-threatening side effects. Nardil, as well as other MAO Inhibitors, prevents a person's liver from metabolizing the enzyme called "Tyramine". Tyramine is found in many foods, such as aged cheese, beer, red wine, sour cream, and some packaged soups. If Tyramine builds up to a high level in a person's blood stream, severe high blood pressure occurs, which can lead to fatal heart attacks and strokes in a matter of an hour or less, if the person goes untreated without medication to lower his blood pressure. For people who do not take Nardil or other MAO Inhibitors, high blood pressure is not a concern, because a person's liver quickly metabolizes the tyramine so that the blood pressure does not increase at all. But for me, a person taking Nardil, it meant a strict avoidance of many foods, such as most cheese pizza, some soups, dips with sour cream, and also certain chemicals, like caffeine and also chocolate, which contains caffeine.

But this restricted diet did not matter, because Nardil was extremely effective against agoraphobia. For the first time since I was 19, I had gone without panic attacks for over a week. I was able to drive expressways again, to eat in restaurants again, to be at peace during the day, and sleep well at night. Dr. Cocoran also put me on Stelazine to take care of the anxiety associated with agoraphobia. However, I was unable to work, because I was still very limited to places where I could go. The agoraphobia was better, but it was still there. I still have a bad fear of elevators, and since most of the job opportunities were in the city in tall buildings, I could not find work. I had to go on disability and I received $200.00 per month from the state. This was one of the hardest things I ever had to do, because I was always a very proud person, and to me this was a humiliating, degrading experience.

But worse than this was the loneliness. All of my friends had graduated from college and were working in good jobs. This meant I did not get a chance to see them very often, and because of not having a job and people to work with everyday, I felt very much alone. One day I was reading the Bible and came across a passage, which was difficult for me to understand. I called up my parish rectory and spoke to Fr. Lany, a priest I had heard at mass the previous Sunday. As it turns out he was extremely friendly, and even though he was 30, he had two Master's Degrees, one in Philosophy and the other in Psychology. He was a brilliant man, and because of his kindness to me, we became good friends very quickly. He explained to me many difficult passages in the Scriptures, which I had struggled with for years, and that removed a lot of psychological depression and anxiety that I had. He had worked in hospitals in the psychiatric wards, and he noticed one thing, which was common to a lot of mentally ill people. He hit the nail right on the head when he said it was lack of trust in God. I knew I didn't trust God the years I had suffered panic attacks. Fr. Lany asked me, "Would a loving Father who became man in the person of Jesus Christ, who died on the cross for me, let gravity stop so I would float off into space alone?" Of course not! Jesus said that "fear is useless, what is needed is trust in God". How true that is, and Fr. Lany pointed that out to me.

Over the next five years, I would make invaluable friendships with priests. I began to go to the Sacrament of Reconciliation face to face sometimes as often as twice a week. I became closer to Jesus and started to develop a personal friendship with my Savior, Lord and Friend. I still was unable to find work, except for part-time as a telephone solicitor, because that was the only job that did not require a four-year degree and make me fill out a formal application for employment, and then try to explain the gaps in my education and why I was not working full-time for years. In order to get a decent job, I knew I needed to get my degree, and toward the end of 1982, I finally pleaded with the Catholic University I had attended in the past to help me get my degree. I told them that for entry-level jobs, the companies require a degree, and said I would get hired once I completed my studies. For lower paying jobs, the companies said I was over qualified. It was a catch 22 situation. The only way I could get a decent job was to get my college degree, but in order to complete my college degree, I needed to have a job paying me money so I could do it.

The people at the Catholic University were extremely helpful, and allowed me to take three tests on a pass/fail basis to complete my remaining general education requirements, and allowed me to take my final management course at home to complete my business school requirements. Finally, in February of 1983, at the age of 28, I received my Bachelor's degree, with a Finance major and a 3.75 out of 4.0 GPA in my major, 11 years after I first started college in 1972.

Unfortunately, it was almost impossible for me to find a decent job due to the economy and to my agoraphobia. I started playing pool in bars for money and I was good at it, so I was able to win enough for a little extra spending money. However, I was drinking alcohol (not beer because I was on Nardil, but rather vodka) and I started to become a pool-shooting bum who was wasting the best years of his life. These were the years a man 25-30 years old gets married and has a family, but due to my handicap, the agoraphobia, it appeared I was destined to be alone for the rest of my life, without at least even a wife, let alone children.

Then, at the age of 29, I met Mary. I was with a friend at a Catholic dance held at a hotel on the northwest side of the city, and I noticed a beautiful blonde, about 5'4" with a perfect figure, dancing with a man on the dance floor. She came back to sit down at the table where I was sitting, and our eyes met. For me, it was love at first sight, and I asked her to dance. I was hoping the dance would never end, because with Mary I felt safe, I felt loved, even though we had just met. After the dance, we went back to the table and talked, and she revealed to me that she was a Christian, not a Catholic as I was, but a nondenominational Christian. She seemed to like me, and the fact that I was a Christian and loved Jesus made me attractive to her. I asked her for a date, and she gave me her phone number. However, when I called the number a few days later, the person who answered said there was no Mary who lived there. I thought it was very cruel for her to give me the wrong number, especially since she said she was a Christian. I thought I would never see her again, and that saddened me greatly.

But, the following Wednesday, a friend of mine who was becoming a priest invited me to a prayer service at a local church. I went with him and when I got there, I saw Mary! I waited until the meeting was over and everyone was socializing, and I approached Mary and asked her why she gave me the wrong number. She told me that she had only been living at her new address for only two weeks, and asked me what number she gave me. When I told her, she then said that was the wrong number, and she then gave me her correct number. As it turns out, she thought I was making up the part about her giving me the wrong number because I really didn't want to go out with her. Thankfully, everything was a mistake, and I realized that she liked me as much as I liked her. I called her again, at the correct number, and we went out on a date at the end of the week.

On the date, when I mentioned that I had agoraphobia, she had never heard of it, and asked me what it was. I explained it briefly to her, and she was very compassionate and understanding. I was afraid it would turn her off, but instead she became closer to me. On our next date, she brought along a little book on agoraphobia. She said that she was reading the book so she could understand my condition better, and possibly help me with it. I could not believe it. I had actually found a woman who accepted me as myself, and didn't care if I was mentally handicapped. She was very special, and she was like an angel sent from God to be my special and closest friend. Again "Fear is useless, what is needed is trust in God". How true I found this to be, time and time again.

Mary and I fell in love, but before we could get married I had to find a full-time job, which paid well enough to enable us to be married. For months my job search proved fruitless. But, then in May of 1984, I landed a job in inside sales with a fortune 500 company, near enough to my home so that I didn't have to worry about agoraphobia. The only problem was that I had to go into the city to the 10th floor of an office building for two weeks to train for the position. Nardil controlled the agoraphobia pretty well, but not well enough for me to handle spending two weeks in the city in a high-rise building. I called Dr. Cocoran and told him my predicament. He suggested a new medication for agoraphobia, which had just recently been approved by the Food and Drug Administration. It was called Ludiomil. He said if I wanted to try it I would first have to stop taking Nardil and

24

Stelazine, and then in a week or two I could start taking Ludiomil. I was scheduled to start work in about a month, toward the end of June, so a week later I stopped taking Nardil and Stelazine. After about a week, I started feeling very depressed and I had tremendous anxiety. I knew I was slipping backwards, but I wanted that job, so I continued to stay off the Nardil and Stelazine, waiting to try the Ludiomil.

I was so incoherent after two weeks that I got confused and started to slip backwards into depression, and to lose weight. I was at the point of despair, because I knew I would have to be hospitalized again, and that I would lose my opportunity for the job, and worst of all, I thought I would lose Mary. I decided in my frenzied state of mind that I wanted to die, so I nervously called my internist, Dr. Kelly, and had him call in a prescription of valium to my pharmacy. In a daze I walked to the pharmacy, picked up the valium, and walked home. I went into my mother's purse, took out her bottle of heart medication, took my bottle of valium and the heart medication into the bathroom and swallowed both entire bottles. I went out into the kitchen immediately and yelled to my parents "I did, I did it", then locked myself in my room and started praying, "Jesus forgive me, Jesus forgive me", over and over again. My parents immediately called 911 and an ambulance was there in what seemed like no time at all. I started to go unconscious as they took me to the local hospital. I found out later they gave me Narcan, a drug used to prevent damage from drug overdoses. That's probably what saved my life, in addition to having my stomach pumped at the hospital and having charcoal shot into my stomach to soak up the valium and heart medication that was still in my gastrointestinal tract, and to prevent it from getting into my bloodstream. As you can tell, I recovered, but I spent the night in intensive care. Mary and my dad spent the entire night in my room with me, and did not sleep at all. The next day, when I was out of physical danger, I was taken by ambulance to the teaching hospital in the city, where I was involuntarily admitted to the psychiatric ward. It was July 4, 1984, and it was the worst day of my life.

Chapter 5

"Even though I walk through the dark valley, I fear no evil; for you are at my side with your rod and staff that give me courage"- Psalm 23:4

This was the second time I was hospitalized in the psychiatric ward but this time I was on a different floor because I had tried to kill myself. It was the floor reserved for people with the most severe psychiatric problems. This floor was like hell to me but I knew that it was where I needed to be. Due to the overdose, I was very depressed and had a paranoid fear of everyone. While I suffered no serious physical damage, I had damaged myself spiritually and psychologically. Dr. Cocoran asked me why I tried to kill myself. I just told him I wanted to be in Heaven, and I wasn't thinking straight, so I tried to kill myself. He answered me by saying, "Well, you won't get to Heaven that way". It's probably true, but, objectively what I did was a serious sin. Take it from me, suicide is not worth it. If you fail, which happens a lot, you risk living the rest of your life in a state worse than before you tried to kill yourself, sometime in a state even worse than death. I could have very easily suffered permanent brain or heart damage from my overdose. If you are successful with your suicide, you destroy God's most precious gift of life. And look at all the people you hurt. Your parents suffer the death of a child, which can cripple them with grief, and fill the rest of their lives with sadness. The same is true for your spouse, and your brothers and sisters, and friends. When you kill yourself, you are not the only victim, you make all your loved ones victims too.

Dr. Cocoran started my treatment by putting me back on Nardil. He chose Nardil because it worked well for me before. I was to spend five weeks in the hospital, he told me, and that my prognosis looked good. The next five weeks went well, largely in part to one of the staff members whose name was Buddy. Buddy was a huge black man in his late 30's, who was married and lived in a suburb of the city. He was 6'4" and about 350 pounds, and he looked a little bit like an ex-football star. Buddy was very intelligent, a devout Christian, and one of the nicest people you could ever meet. His size was intimidating, but he was one of the kindest men on the face of the earth. Indeed, he was a "gentle giant". He reached out in friendship to me, and we became quick friends. We played bingo and chess almost every day, and had many talks about God. Seeing Buddy five days a week made the next 5 weeks go a little easier for me.

Also, Mary, my mom, dad and my brother John came to see me often, and I knew I was loved. I regretted my act of attempted suicide even more now, because I realized they would have been incomplete without me around, and that I would have robbed them of someone very dear to them if I had been successful in killing myself. If you feel suicidal, go immediately to the best hospital's emergency room. Seek help, not death.

In late August of 1984, I was released and went home to live with my parents. I was still depressed and I could not function very well. This went on for months and in the beginning of December of 1984, Dr. Cocoran hospitalized me again, for the 3rd time, with severe depression and high levels of anxiety. I was so out of it that I had even forgotten how to dress myself after taking a shower. Here was a 30-year-old man with a high IQ and I was reduced to a vegetable. But Jesus never left my side. He was allowing all this to happen so he could remake me from the ground up. I had to die to my old self in order to become the person Jesus wanted me to be. In the Gospel Jesus says that, "Unless a seed falls to the ground and dies, it cannot bear fruit". This was what was occurring with me.

For the first three weeks it looked as if I might have to spend the rest of my life in state mental hospitals, because my condition was that serious. Then Dr. Cocoran consulted with another psychiatrist and they put their heads together to see what could be done. They put me on new medications, Loxitane and Tegretol, and in a few days I regained my mind. Dr. Cocoran then put me on Ludiomil for my agoraphobia and it was as if I had been reborn. I now had the beginning of a new life, one filled with faith, hope and love. I look back now, and see the loving hand of God restoring me back to health. It was a week before Christmas, 1984, and things were looking up.

Also, Mary was a jewel, a true gift from God to me. She never abandoned me, and prayed for me constantly. She visited me on Christmas day, and when she saw me she started to cry. I comforted her by telling her I loved her and that things would be okay. She did not want to give me up, even though I thought she would probably be better off without me. I had no job, and the prospects of getting a job looked very slim. So I told her she should try to forget me, and try to find someone else. But she never did.

Then a startling discovery was made. While in the hospital I had been complaining of chest pains quite a lot, since I no longer had the anxiety level I had when I first came in, Dr. Kelly, my internist, decided to check things out further. He suspected I had problems with my esophagus, so he called in a gastroenterologist. To my surprise the gastroenterologist, Dr. Hamilton, listened to my heart first, and told me that my chest pain was being caused by my heart. He told me I had a mitral valve prolapse, a heart murmur which is not serious, but which causes severe chest pain, shortness of breath, dizziness, neck, shoulder, or back pain, and which can make you feel like you're dying. He said the symptoms of a mitral valve prolapse mimic those of a heart attack, but they also mimic those of a panic attack! He told me that my mitral valve prolapse was very mild, and that it had remained undetected for all my life, because you have to listen to the heart in a special way to detect it. In reality, he said, you have to be looking for it to find it, and since I had the agoraphobia, everyone assumed that the chest pains were due to panic attacks. A subsequent echocardiogram revealed that in fact Dr. Hamilton's diagnosis would be correct. I did have a borderline mitral valve prolapse. So I was right, he told me, that when I was 19, the first "panic" attack I had was actually a mitral valve prolapse attack. This was astonishing news! Dr. Cocoran agreed with Dr. Hamilton that many times so-called panic attacks are actually being caused by a mitral valve prolapse, but the results can be the same, namely crippling anxiety. Dr. Cocoran told me that if I had known about the mitral valve prolapse when I was 19, I probably would not have developed agoraphobia and panic disorder. Some of my panic attacks were mitral valve prolapse attacks, but most of them were really just panic attacks themselves, due to the fear I expressed at the age of 19.

Just the knowledge of identifying the mitral valve prolapse relieved a lot of anxiety. I could not die from the prolapse, and if my mitral valve acted up, I should just sit down and wait for the chest pain, or shortness of breath, dizziness, or other symptoms, or combination of all, to go away.

Armed with this new knowledge, I was ready to start my new life. I was released from the hospital in January 1985. I was not arrogant anymore, for I had been humbled by my condition and realized that I owed everything to God. Now I would live my life for the Lord, and I knew that He would not let me down. I had experienced the mighty, loving hand of Jesus Christ, and I knew that He would always be with me, no matter where I am. Yes, even in the hell of a psychiatric ward, Jesus was there, working his miracle on me. I did not fear the future now, for I knew that even if I ended up on the street as one of the homeless, my Lord would always be with me, no matter where I was.

Chapter 6

"Know that I am with you always, until the end of the world"- Matthew 28:20

So, at the age of 30, I had a new lease on life. Shortly after I came home from the hospital, I got in contact with the county agency which was to be in charge of my rehabilitation. For six weeks I was to attend a hospital program during the day in which I would be shown how to maintain a checkbook, cook for myself, and interview for a job. After that I would receive help in obtaining steady employment, and then would live in a group apartment with other people who suffered from mental illness, where my medication would be monitored. However, there was a three month waiting period to get into the program, so I thought I would try to find a job on my own, so I could keep busy until I could be accepted into the program. Also, I already knew how to balance a checkbook, cook for myself, and interview for a job, so I felt it was time to leave the past behind, and take a giant step forward into the future.

I saw an ad in the local paper for a sales position with a local cable television company, and I was able to obtain an interview with the sales manager, whose name was Randy. During the interview I was asked several questions to determine if I was right for the job. I had only some telemarketing experience from years before, so I didn't have high hopes of securing a position with Randy's firm, but I answered the questions honestly and to the best of my ability. My overriding theme in responding to his questions was my faith in Jesus Christ. Randy seemed to be impressed with my honesty and sincerity, and immediately had me talk with the V.P. of sales, Jon. The V.P. of sales probed deeper, but I kept centering on the fact that my faith in Christ would help me to perform the job quite capably and efficiently. Jon asked me if I ever read the Bible, and I mentioned to him that I had been reading and studying the Bible, at that time, for over 11 years. Now Jon was not a religious man, he told me at one point in the interview, but when I told him about my Bible knowledge, his interest in me peaked. He seemed quite impressed with my persuasive abilities and offered me the position on the spot. I accepted immediately, for the job had a very good base salary, plus commission and benefits. I left the interview in a state of joy, and thanked Jesus for getting the job for me. The interview had occurred on Friday and I was to begin work the following Monday.

I started the position not knowing very much about what was being broadcasted on cable T.V., but quickly learned. The job itself required selling door to door, and this didn't bother me until I actually tried doing it. Just about everyone in the neighborhood with whom I spoke was totally uninterested in acquiring cable TV for their home. Firstly because of the cost and secondly because of what was broadcasted on it. R-rated movies being shown on the main cable stations turned off many people to cable TV. Granted there are many fine programs and networks on cable TV, but at that time cable TV was new and by and large these programs were in the minority. I stayed on the position for about a week, and after having frozen hands from walking door to door in freezing weather and dropping off flyers in mailboxes, I was ready to quit. But, here again, God was watching over me. I picked up the local paper, and in the job section I saw a large ad, which read "FINANCE SALES". It was an ad for a broker position with a mortgage brokerage firm located two miles from my home, called ABCD Mortgage Company. I called the company and talked to the V.P. of the company, a man called Rick. Rick was impressed with my degree and my presentation and called me in for an interview. Another miracle was about to begin.

The next day I met a man about my own age named Norbert. Norbert was the sales manager. He was a nice man, very friendly and with a good sense of humor. We became good friends almost instantly, and we are still close friends to this day. As it turns out, Norbert used to work with Randy at the same cable TV company for which I was presently working, and that became a great icebreaker for the start of the interview. He mentioned to me that he thought the market for cable TV was already saturated in the territory I was working, and he seemed anxious to tell me about the position ABCD Mortgage Company had to offer. I mentioned again during the interview about my faith in Christ, and Norbert was impressed with my faith and sincerity, even though he, like Jon at the cable TV company, was agnostic. Norbert was sold on my ability to perform the job, and he said I would be called back for a second interview in two days. On the second interview, I, for the first time met Rick, the V.P. Rick was a heavyset man in his late 40's, who was very intelligent, and asked me a lot of tough questions. Rick too was agnostic, but he was impressed, as was Norbert, with my faith in God. To make a long story short, I was hired for the position, and I was to start on Monday. For the first time in my life, I thought I had found the ideal job. See how mysteriously God works. For years I had been looking for the ideal job and here it was, just five minutes away from home. The building was only five stories high, so my agoraphobic fear of elevators would not be present, and Norbert had told me that there would be no traveling. Also, I would have my own office, not a cubical, but an office. It was the perfect job for me, because I would have no agoraphobia to interfere with my work, one where I could settle in and make a career and call home.

Norbert had told me, when I had interviewed with him on Monday, that the hours would be 1pm to 9pm on Monday, Tuesday and Thursday, and 9am to 5pm on Wednesday and Friday. However, when I started work on Monday, Rick told me that the hours would be 9am to 9pm Monday, Tuesday, and Thursday, and 9am to 5pm on Wednesday and Friday, and that once a week I would have to go to the County Recorder of Deeds Office to get leads for work. Also, he showed me my office and it was great, with plenty of room and prestige. I began to panic inside. I could never do the traveling thing on the expressways due to my agoraphobia, and after seeing my office I thought that this job was out of my league, that I would never be capable of keeping it. The next chance I had to talk to Rick in private, I tried to bow out from the job gracefully. He asked me why, and said he really

36

wanted me to stay. I told him about the agoraphobia and the inability to travel, and that I thought the job, along with the hours, three 12-hour days per week, would be too much for me to handle.

He kept trying to convince me to stay, but I kept saying no. Finally, he went into another office to talk to Hank, the President. Hank was a tall man in his late 40's and by the way he dressed I could tell he was a millionaire. Hank called me into his office and politely invited me to have a seat. I started to explain why I didn't think I could do the job, but he put his hand out with his palm up for me to stop talking, and said he didn't care about that. He worked up some numbers on his calculator and told me that if I would get six loans per month, I would make $20,000.00 per year, not including bonuses, which, in 1985, was a good income. He also told me that if I wanted to work part-time and stay part-time, that was fine with him. If I wanted to start part-time and then wanted to go full-time, I could do that also, and if I felt that full-time work was too much for me, I could go back to part-time hours and stay part-time. Or else, he said, I could start full-time and stay full-time with the hours being 1pm to 9pm three days a week, and 9am to 5pm on Wednesday and Friday, and that I would never have to leave the office if I didn't want to. Hank took all the pressure off me, because he saw potential in me, which I didn't see in myself. Hank was Jewish, and had a deep respect for God and his fellow man, and he treated me with kindness and respect.

I started work that day, and I liked the job tremendously. I even worked the following Saturday, I was so interested in my work. Hank called and talked to me on Saturday to encourage me and tell me I was doing a great job. Again, all I can say is that God is a good God, and never stops watching after His children. After three months at ABCD Mortgage Company, I became the top producer in the office, and made much more money than what Hank had estimated on his calculator tape that day of my interview. After I had been with ABCD Mortgage Company for three years, I received a special compensation package from Hank, which increased my income by 70%. But more importantly, this position had been the longest lasting position I had ever held. I have been with ABCD now for 18 years, and I still find the job as interesting and exciting as the day I first started. Last year, in 1996, I made $65,000.00. And, too, I have never lost my gratitude and love for Hank, who has become more than my boss, he became my close friend.

During the next five years I made great strides in dealing with my agoraphobia. In 1986, I drove 100 miles to a popular resort in a neighboring state, for a weekend, something I never would have been able to do before then. I owe a lot of my accomplishment in conquering my agoraphobia to Mary, who has been at my side, faithfully, for the last 20 years. However, four years ago, the panic attacks started again. I became afraid to go to work, and sometimes, to even venture outside the house. I was regressing and I knew, if I continued, I would need to quit work. Fortunately, God had other plans for me. Agoraphobia had made its final onslaught against me, but Jesus took care of it for good. Thank God for Dr. Cocoran. He put me on what was then a new drug called Klonopin, which worked better than any medication I had taken in the past, and within a day I was able to function normally again. Also, roughly two years ago, my antidepressant was switched from Ludiomil to Zoloft, which also helps control panic disorder with agoraphobia. My Lord never leaves me. I am doing things now that I never thought I would be able to do.

In this book earlier I had mentioned how God only permits evil so that a greater good will come of it. I would like to give you some examples of how this was true in my life.

First, there's the case of my mom. My mom had heart trouble since 1971, when she suffered a heart attack. At one point, a local doctor had put her on a heart medication, and was not very familiar with the drug. At one point, he wanted her to stop taking it because it precipitated asthma for her, and he told her to stop taking the heart medication cold turkey. I was concerned about this and called my internist, Dr. Kelly, at the teaching hospital in the City for his advice. He told me if she stopped taking the heart medication without weaning off the drug gradually, she could have another heart attack and die. He talked to my mom on the phone and told her how to wean off the drug gradually over a three-week period, to prevent any danger to her heart or her life. In other words, he probably saved her life. My mom was put under the care of a cardiologist, who was part of a group of cardiologists from the teaching hospital in the City, and she received excellent care. This would not have occurred had I not met Dr. Kelly when I was hospitalized for agoraphobia in the teaching hospital in the City. Also, my brother's life was recently saved. He suffered a heart attack four years ago, and it was the same cardiologist that my mom saw, who saved his life in the emergency room.

In regard to Dr. Cocoran, he has helped many people I know. I referred my friend Rob, a friend from our parish, who had severe anxiety and suffered from spastic colon as the result of it. Dr. Cocoran put him on Klonopin, the same medication I take, and he did fine. However, in 1997, at the age of 63, he recently passed away due to liver cancer, and I miss him a lot. (Cancer runs in his family; it was not due to the Klonopin.) My friend Mark, who is a recovering alcoholic, found out after he became sober that he suffered from depression. After seeing a local psychiatrist who didn't know how to treat him, Mark went to see Dr. Cocoran at my suggestion. Mark is now quite happy and normal, and is doing fine. Mark got married eight years ago and I was his best man. Mary's friend from her company had a husband who was suffering from panic attacks and was at the point where he could no longer do his work.

I referred him to Dr. Cocoran, who put him on medication and he is now doing fine. Also, as for my brother, after he had his heart attack and almost died, he started suffering from panic attacks also, due to his brush with death. He started seeing Dr. Cocoran, was put on medication, and is coming back to normality, with much less fear in his life. My brother recently moved out of state with his fiancé and is doing well. So as you can see, all things do work together for the good for those who love God.

Chapter 7

"Be therefore wise as serpents, and innocent as doves"- Matthew 10:16

It was not easy writing this book. It brought back many painful memories for me. But if just one person who has agoraphobia is helped by my suffering, it will all be worth it, because I would not want anyone to go through what I did. I am one of the fortunate ones. I have been given a great gift from God. The gift of a second mind. I believe I survived my suicide attempt because God knew I would need to help other people who are suffering too, and in this book I have attempted to do just that. Things are not easy for me. I still have agoraphobia, and even though it is at a much lower degree, I still have my bad days. I still have problems with shopping malls and driving some expressways, but my job has not suffered because of it. God has been very good to me. If I did not have agoraphobia, I would never have met Mary, who I have been married to for eight years. In 1985, I would never have believed I could ever get a woman to even like me, let alone love me, but Mary has done just that. I thank God for the gift of her. Also, ABCD Mortgage Company allows me to work from an office at my home. I have been working from home for almost one and a half years now, and it is very convenient - I have almost no panic attacks.

I would like to throw in some advice as I complete this book. Dr. Cocoran says that one study estimated that as many as 4.5% of the population routinely suffer from panic disorder. It affects 2-3% of women and 0.5-1.5% of men. The typical age of onset is the mid 20's. It affects women more than men by approximately 2 to 1, half of whom don't know they have it or how to treat it. I would like to make some suggestions if you think you have agoraphobia. First of all, make sure you really do have agoraphobia and not a mitral valve prolapse. The only way you can tell for sure is for a good cardiologist from a leading hospital to examine you. There is a special way to tell if you have a mitral valve prolapse. You must lay flat on your back, bear down as if moving your bowels for 10-15 seconds, then breathe normally as the cardiologist listens to your heart. Dr. Ebert, my cardiologist, a leading expert in mitral valve prolapse, did just that, and discovered I had a grade 1 to 2 murmur. I had an echocardiogram done by Dr. Ebert four years ago, and it found no evidence of a mitral valve prolapse. However, he told me, and this is important, that about 30% of the time, echocardiograms will miss a mitral valve prolapse, even if several echocardiograms are done. The only way to make a sure and certain diagnosis of a mitral valve prolapse, he told me, is by listening to the heart. There is no substitute for a good set of ears. It's important that you know whether or not you have a mitral valve prolapse for several reasons. For one, before you have dental work you should be premedicated with amoxycillin to prevent the risk of contracting bacterial endocarditis, a heart valve infection that can be fatal. The odds of this occurring without being on amoxycillin is only 1 in 2,500, but even so, Dr. Ebert says that you don't want to take even the smallest chance, when a heart valve infection can be prevented so easily with antibiotic prophylaxis. Another reason is that if the mitral valve prolapse is of a more severe type, heart medication can be prescribed to treat it and lessen its symptoms. If you go into psychotherapy assuming you have panic attacks, but really have a mitral valve prolapse, you will suffer needlessly for years as I did, because psychiatrists and psychologists, as a rule, are not familiar with heart problems. Also, a mitral valve prolapse is almost never fatal. The odds of dying from it are about a million to one, Dr. Ebert says. Knowing that you won't die from a mitral valve prolapse attack can give you a lot of peace of mind. I know that to be true in my case, because when my mitral valve prolapse acts up, it does feel like I am going to die, and knowing that I won't die keeps me from panicking. And yes, I can now distinguish between a mitral valve prolapse attack and a panic attack, and you know what, I get hardly any panic attacks these days as long as I avoid very open spaces. Second, if it's determined by a good cardiologist, from a teaching hospital, that you do not have a mitral valve prolapse or any other heart problems, then see a good psychiatrist not a psychologist. A psychologist is not an M.D., and cannot prescribe medication. Only a psychiatrist can prescribe medication, and take it from me, you can talk about panic attacks until you are blue in the face, but that won't help you one bit. Only the right medication or medications can control panic attacks, and help relieve your suffering, accompanied by psychotherapy. Only a psychiatrist can prescribe medication, a psychologist can't, but most importantly, if at all possible, get under the care of a psychiatrist from a teaching hospital, because teaching hospitals are by and large where the best psychiatrists are. If you can avoid it, stay away from psychiatrists who belong to community hospitals or to totally psychiatric institutions, or else you could get stuck with a psychiatrist like Dr. Lupek, as I did, and suffer needlessly for years.

Third, if you have agoraphobia with panic disorder, don't give up. There are numerous medications on the market today to treat panic disorder, and in the future there will be more, so don't fall into despair. God is a <u>loving</u> God, and if you seek Him above all else, He will <u>never</u> let you down. Isaiah says, "Can a mother forget her children, the child of her womb? Even should she forget, I will never forget you." In Jesus Christ we have a sure and certain hope of Eternal life, of Eternal happiness, and any suffering we endure on this earth is worth it, because Heaven is worth it. This life is temporary, Heaven is eternal, and we must always keep our focus on that truth. But God won't let you be tested beyond your strength. Saint Paul assures us that with each temptation God will give us a way to endure it. So keep your faith strong, knowing that if your faith is a persistent faith and if you ask God to heal you, He <u>will</u> heal you. It may not be the healing you expect, or the healing you think would be the best for you, but you will receive a healing nonetheless.

Fourth, realize that you have a handicap, and that even though a handicap puts limits on what you can do, it does not prevent you from leading a relatively full life. One thing most agoraphobics don't realize is that they can get a handicapped parking card to allow them to park in the handicapped parking spaces at shopping centers, movie theaters, or any other place where there is a handicapped parking space. Panic disorder is classified as a legitimate handicap, just as if you were in a wheelchair, and entitles you to handicapped parking privileges. I have found that this greatly increases my ability to do shopping, go to the movies, and do many other things I otherwise would not be able to do if I did not have a handicapped-parking card.

Fifth, try to get affordable health insurance, without going on public aid if you can avoid it. Through an insurance broker I know, according to him, the State of Illinois offers an insurance policy for people who are uninsurable under any other plan, called the Illinois Comprehensive Health Insurance Plan, or ICHIP for short. ICHIP offers a deductible of $500, $1,000 or $1,500 and a $2,000 maximum out-of-pocket expense per year, and the premiums are only 30% higher than a standard health insurance policy. If you live in Illinois, call the State of Illinois to find out more about it. If you live outside Illinois, check to see if your state offers a similar health insurance plan. There is usually a three to six month waiting period before you can be enrolled, but it is well worth the wait. Usually public aid does not give you access to the best medical care, but ICHIP and other policies like it, will give you access to doctors and hospitals of higher caliber.

Finally, good can come out of agoraphobia. If it were not for agoraphobia, I would not have the job I love and for which I am most suited. I probably would never have met Mary, my mother and brother could very well have died, my friends would be suffering, and I would not be as close to Christ as I am today. By having agoraphobia with panic disorder, I have lost my arrogance and pride which I had before I contracted agoraphobia. I have learned to rely totally on God, to let God be in control, and the paradox of it all is that the less I'm in control, the more control over my life God gives me. Right now, I'm doing fine, where I'll end up only God knows. But I face the future full of confidence now, and I know that whatever happens to me, God has a reason for it. I may not know that reason in this life, but I will in the next. I know that Jesus Christ died on the cross for me because He loves me, and that He wants me to be happy, and that my Friend and True Love is in Heaven. Life is simple: we come from God, we return to God for all Eternity.

I thank God for my agoraphobia because so many good things came out of it, so many people have been touched by Jesus because of it. Yes, there is sadness and pain with agoraphobia, the panic attacks are terrible, but we all have our crosses to bear in this life. But Christ also says to us all, "Come to me you who are heavy burden, and I will give you rest, for my yoke is easy, and my burden is light". The biggest fear for an agoraphobic is often fear of death, because I know when I have a panic attack it feels like I'm going to die. But when you have Jesus, death is no longer an enemy to be feared. Yes, with Jesus we die, but with Jesus we also rise again. As St. Paul says, "Death, where is your victory, death, where is your sting?" Death is an enemy that Jesus has already conquered for us over 2000 years ago. In closing, I would hope that my story would help those with panic disorder. I know that my story is not unique, and that what happened to me is happening to millions of people as I write. For those who have panic disorder, and who feel that it is unbearable, keep hope, keep your trust in God. This life is only temporary, and your condition will pass. Eventually our home is in Heaven with Jesus; keep your focus on that fact. Keep your focus on that truth, because God loves you and has prepared for you a place in Heaven. Thank you, Jesus. May God bless everyone who reads this book.

About the Author

Michael R. Patrick was born in the Midwest and then he and his family moved to another state due to his father's transfer for work. He lived there for 4 years, and then moved back to the Midwest area, he attended a Catholic High School and went to DePaul University to study business. He excelled at virtually all his courses and ended up graduating "Summa Cum Laude" with a 3.62/4.0 G.P.A overall, a 3.75/4.0 G.P.A. in his major, which was finance, and a 4.0/4.0 G.P.A. in his minor which was Management. DePaul also wanted to sponsor him for the Rhodes Scholarship, but he turned it down because he did not want to go to Europe to study. He leads an excellent job as a mortgage broker, and he still does some on a semi-retired basis, making-writing books to become closer to God. To Michael, God alone matters, and it is only God who Michael wants to please.